Natural Skin and Body Care

Keeping Your Skin Healthy

Natural Health/Beauty Series

Dueep J. Singh

Mendon Cottage Books

JD-Biz Publishing

Disclaimer

The information is this book is provided for informational purposes only. It is not intended to be used and medical advice or a substitute for proper medical treatment by a qualified health care provider. The information is believed to be accurate as presented based on research by the author.

The contents have not been evaluated by the U.S. Food and Drug Administration or any other Government or Health Organization and the contents in this book are not to be used to treat cure or prevent disease.

The author or publisher is not responsible for the use or safety of any diet, procedure or treatment mentioned in this book. The author or publisher is not responsible for errors or omissions that may exist.

Warning

The Book is for informational purposes only and before taking on any diet, treatment or medical procedure, it is recommended to consult with your primary health care provider.

Check out some of the other Healthy Gardening Series books at Amazon.com

Gardening Series on Amazon

Check out some of the other Health Learning Series books at Amazon.com

Health Learning Series on Amazon

Table of Contents

Introduction

Have you noticed that everybody who is self-conscious and beauty conscious is very careful about applying makeup, which focuses on the face, but they do not bother much about skin and body care for the rest of the body?

That is the reason why you may have skin tones, a shade or two lighter than the rest of your body because you have been bleaching it or slathering sunscreen lotion on it.

Just go into the shower and do a careful survey of the rest of your body. You are going to be surprised to see parts of it which have been neglected for ages. In fact, let me admit it. I find rubbing and scrubbing the lower extremities below the knee, a big bore, because I have to bend over so much, to get to my knees, ankles and feet. Even sitting down and lifting them up in order to scrub them is a major headache. You may think this reason so absurd. According to me, I think it perfectly reasonable!

Believe it or not, most of us have some silly excuse or reason to justify why we neglect major portions of our body, so much. That is why we have rough elbows and rough knees and perhaps neglected feet, especially the dead cells around the soles and so on.

So this book is going to tell you many natural skin and body care tips and techniques, which you can use easily on your body. Remember your face may be your fortune, but the rest of your body is equally important. So remember to cherish it.

Knowing More about Your Skin

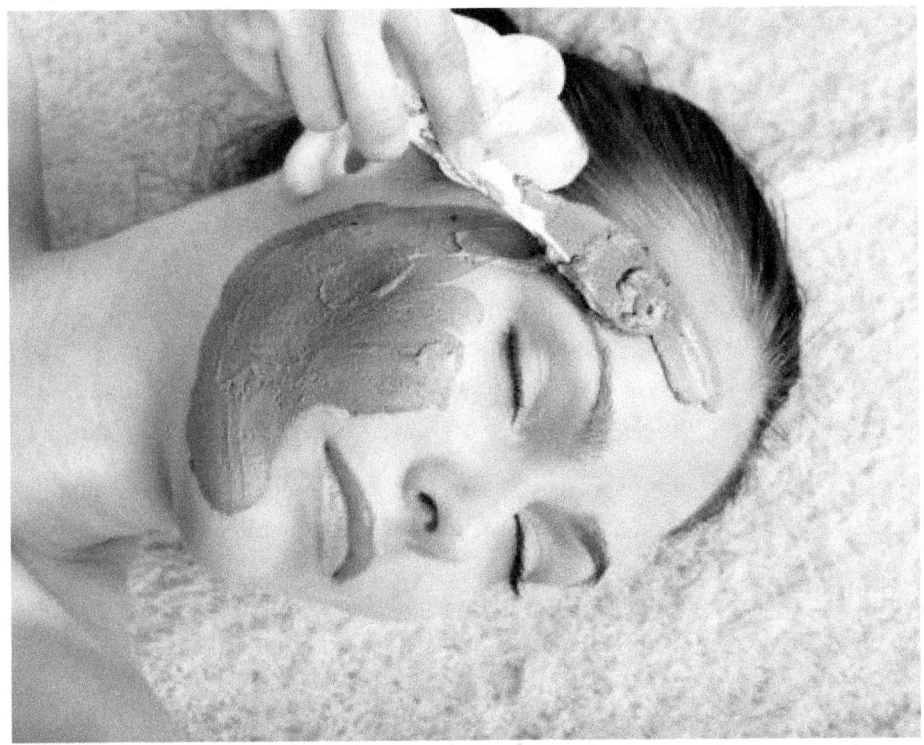

Your skin is a very complicated organ. It is your first line of defense against infection. It has millions of nerve endings to provide you with a sense of touch. It is strong, sensitive and flexible. It is also capable of excreting waste products and oils.

The texture of your skin is definitely going to add to the first impression one gets about you. It was said about Georgiana, the Duchess of Devonshire in Regency times that the reason why she was considered to be such a beauty was because she had perfect porcelain, flawless skin. Her face was like that of a smooth Dresden China doll. Until Beau Brummell, the arbitrator of fashion at that time said, "the known beauties of our age are very lovely in face and form. However, the rest of their bodies are greasy, grimy and dirty."

In fact, he brought in the trend of regular bathing once a day and made it fashionable. This was when he persuaded the Prince Regent to have a bath so that one could see what he looked like under the dirt. And so bathing became the rule instead of the exception. Until then bathing was definitely not fashionable, both among aristocrats and the common people for centuries. According to them, water harmed the skin and that is why *they never bathed.*

One can just imagine going into an atmosphere full of stinking bodies, but I guess all of them had gotten inured to the assault to their nostrils. Instead, they drenched their bodies with perfume.

It is said about fastidious Queen Margot [Margaret of Valois the youngest daughter of Catherine de Medici] who got married to Henry III of Navarre, that she requested her new bridegroom to at least wash his feet, if not take a bath before the marriage was consummated. In answer, he said that he did not intend to do anything so abhorrent and effeminate. Real men did not bathe. No wonder the marriage was annulled.

So, talking about our skin, and why we need to keep it clean ;we know that the skin remains soft by continually renewing itself, and by self-lubrication. A healthy skin is going to have a slightly acidic pH balance. It also secretes antimicrobial substances which are going to help to maintain a poor president balance of friendly microorganisms.

However, is destined grime are allowed to accumulate on the surface of the skin, it is going to give rise to many skin problems, including pimples. An unhealthy skin is the clearest sign of possible ill health.

The accumulation of toxins in your body is going to make your skin look shallow, dry and without luster. On the other hand, if you have a healthy, and hydrated system you are going to have a rich and glowing skin. That is the reason why any dehydration symptoms are going to show up by drying out your skin first.

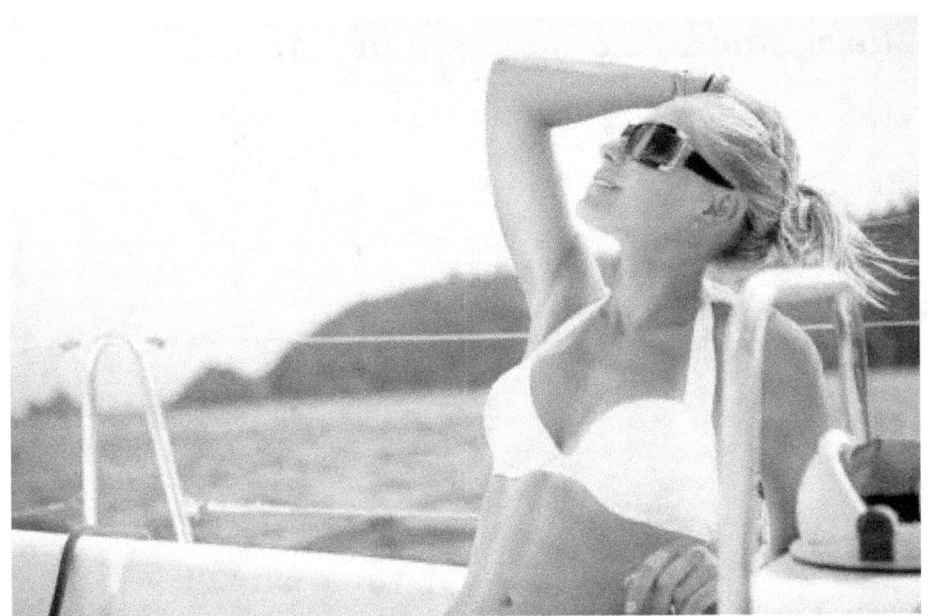

Sun worshiping is all very fine, but it is going to have already disastrous effect on your skin, in the long run. You are going to have dry skin more prone to wrinkles.

Natural Skincare Products in the Market

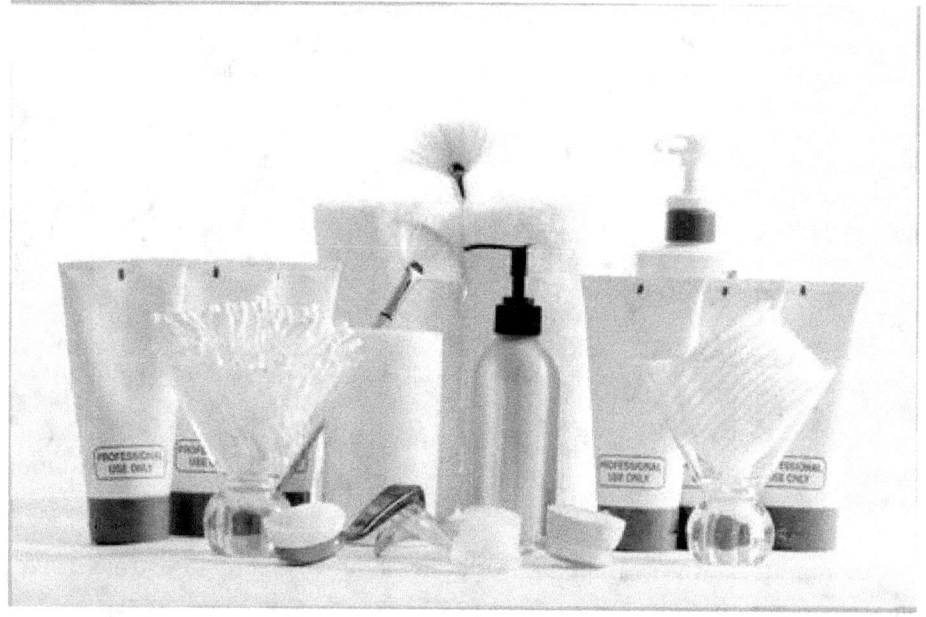

These may be marketed as natural beauty products, but in most cases, they are just a mixture of chemical ingredients.

There are many brands in the market, touting their products as hundred percent natural. Just look at the ingredients used in the products. You are going to be surprised to see that just one or two items are "natural", while the rest of them are chemical fillers and preservers.

A really natural product is definitely not going to have any sort of artificial chemical, including colorings. And also, the shelf life of this product is going to be comparatively less, because it does not have preservatives added to it. That is the reason why any beauty product which you make at home is immediately put in the fridge, is not it.

Making your own beauty products mean that the products are pure, and there are no additives or preservatives that may irritate your skin. Make sure that you buy the highest quality ingredients you can afford, or get those items straight from your garden. At least then you know that you are buying something of top quality or using something which you know is absolutely pure.

Some of the best natural in gradients out there, include oatmeal, honey, milk, fresh fruit juices and fruit pulp, eggs, China Clay etc.. These items have been used for centuries to clean and nourish the skin.

Traditional Oatmeal wash

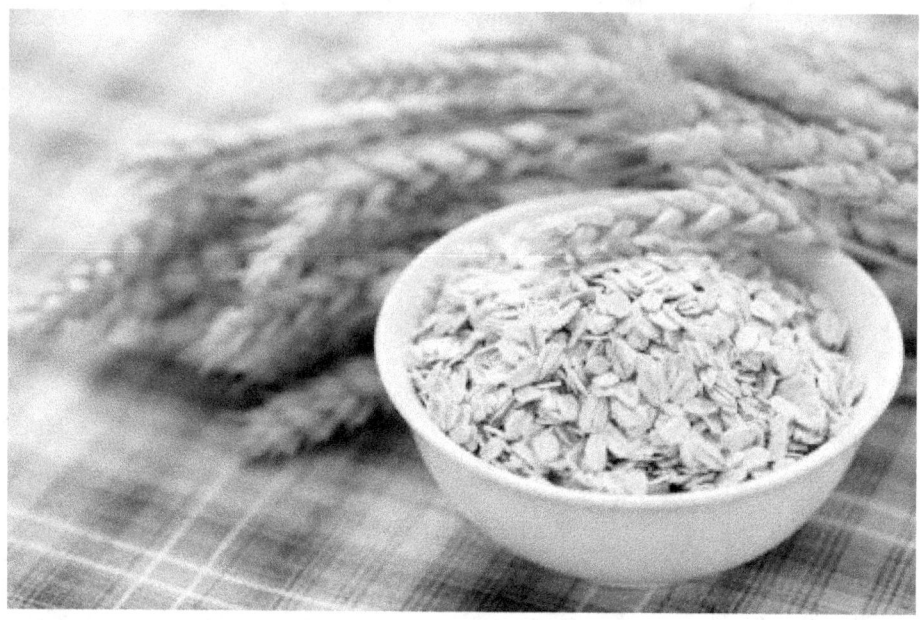

Oatmeal is a healthy cereal, as well as an excellent beauty product.

In Asia, traditional washes are normally made up of rice flour or gram flour, which is gritty, and an excellent base for other cleansing agents. However, oatmeal is equally good or even better, because it is excellent for delicate and sensitive skin. It is also good for curing irritable and inflamed skin conditions.

If you do not have oatmeal around handy, you can always use wheat bran. It is equally gritty, and equally effective. Actually, you need some flour/bran as a gritty solid powdery base to which any liquid is added before you can apply the paste as a cleansing agent on your skin.

So, you can now make a gritty oat wash, by taking a spoonful of oats, mixing it with half a teaspoonful of wheat bran or rice flour, and one teaspoonful of fine sea salt. Sea salt is extremely invigorating, and restores the pH value of your skin. Make it into a paste with one desert spoonful of vegetable oil. I normally use wheat germ oil, almond oil or coconut oil, because I find they are extremely good moisturizers.

Just take this mixture on the palm of your hand and mix gently with a little bit of warm water. It is going to become milky/creamy, because of the oats. Apply it all over your body in small circular motions, using water, whenever you think the mixture is dry.

Then scrub off, gently, getting rid of all the dust and grime, and enjoy your shower.

In many parts of these, this wash has been used for centuries in lieu of soap. Even today, women in villages in remote parts of Asia who do not want to bother about chemical-based soaps and do not have the time to make their own homemade soaps, use this wash and their skins are smooth, flawless and beautiful.

If you want to preserve this cleansing wash, all you need to do is take 4 dessert spoons full of oats, one teaspoonful of wheat bran or ground rice or gram flour, one teaspoonful of sea salt and your favorite oil. Rub this mixture through your fingers until you reach your preferred texture, consistency. If the oats are really rough, the eventual wash is going to be coarser, so you can either have coarse oats, or oats which are more finely ground. Add the rest of the dry ingredients, as well as your favorite essential oil or your vegetable oil or your preferred oil. Olive oil is also an excellent moisturizer.

Rub. Well, until all the oil has been absorbed into the mixture. Press down firmly into a clean glass jar. This is going to last you for anywhere between one week to 3 weeks, depending how often you use it!

To use this, all you have to do is put the ingredients in the middle of the drawstring bag, and draw the string. Once you are ready to step into the bath, dip the bag into the water, squeeze the oats down to the bottom of the bag and the oat – milk will seep through the pores of the cloth.

You can now use this bag, like a sponge. Rub it all over your body, washing your skin with this milky liquid that seeps through the pores of your wash bag

Use plenty of water to keep the bag soft and the oats, creamy, and damp. Once you feel you are silky smooth and squeaky clean, just throw away all the oats and wash the cloth ready again for your next use.

If you are the DIY type of person, and you also have a seaming machine handy, you can make a really nice drawstring bag out of muslin cloth or out of good quality cotton. Here is one excellent URL, giving you the instructions. Make a small bag, – following the instructions given here.

http://www.youtube.com/watch?v=5A82qJnhPN0

The 2 squares should be made up of natural unbleached cotton cloth or muslin cloth, – which is also known as cheesecloth, – measuring about 45 x 45 cm/18 x 18 inches. This is just about the right measurements which are going to fit right into your hand!

The drawstring ribbon can be anywhere between 40 cm to 60 cm, depending on your choice. I normally take 60 cm – about 2 feet of ribbon, because I like to tie the bag over my back, so that the water can run freely through the bag while my bath tub is filling up with fragrant and soft water. You can use any preferred herbs if you want in order to give yourself for refreshing fragrant and rejuvenating soak. But if you are having a hot shower, you can use the string bag held in your hand like a sponge.

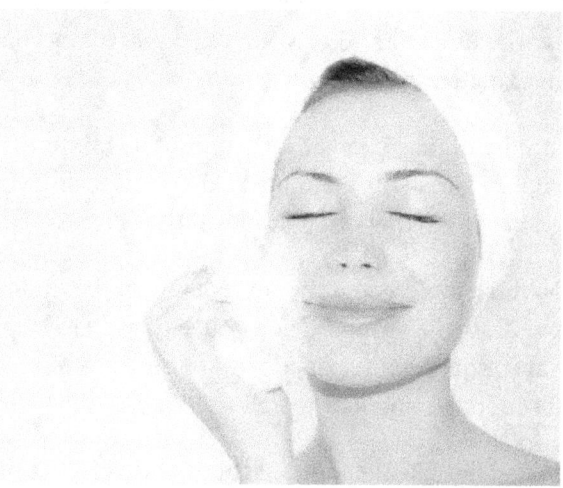

Scrubbing your face and body with an oatmeal scrub is the best way in which you can refresh yourself after a hard day at the office.

In the same way, you can make a wheat bran scrub, which is rather rough, and could take the place of a loofah! For one application you will need 2 tablespoonful of oats, 2 teaspoons full of fine salt, 2 table spoons full of wheat bran and 2 teaspoons full of your favorite oil.

A friend told me that she used dried thyme as a scrub herb in order to break down cellulite. You can also use rosemary, especially in the winter because it stimulates the circulation.

Blend all these ingredients together and thoroughly.

To use, take a handful of this mixture in your cloth bag or in the hand and rub into the skin using a circular rubbing motion. Brush it off, when you think that the oil has seeped into your skin. This is excellent for removing dead skin and stimulating the circulation. This is also good for the drainage of your lymph glands. That means the body is getting rid of toxins, especially through the skin and bringing a healthy glow to it.

Getting Rid of Wrinkles

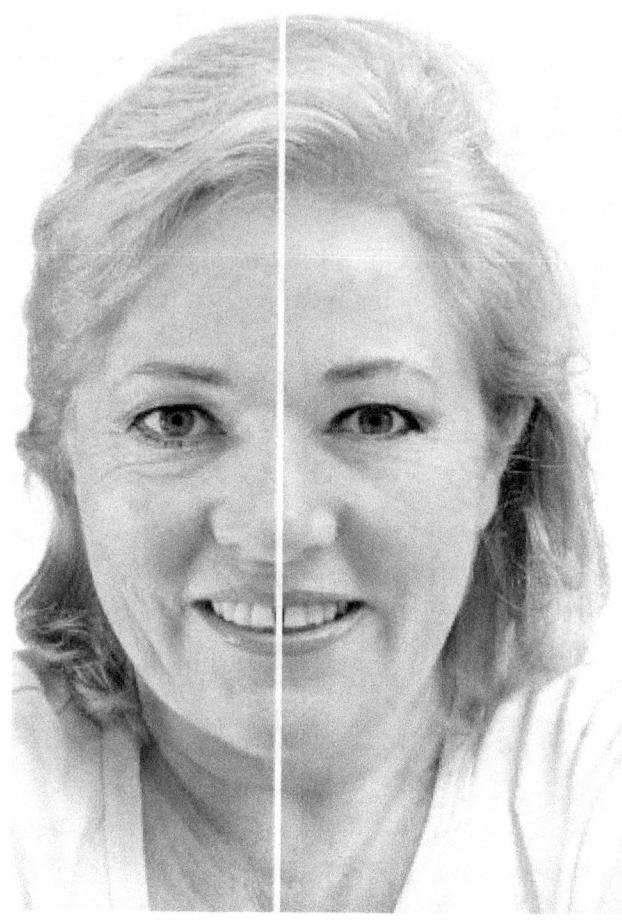

Wrinkles do not have to be a worrisome part of your life, when you reach your 50s and 60s. That is when you use natural remedies to take care of these wrinkles.

Many of my friends are surprised, when they see my skin, which is absolutely wrinkle free. According to them, that is not fair, because anybody who will never see 45 again should at least show Crow feet, wrinkles or even some lines on the face and around the neck.

In fact, a cosmetic company asked me whether I would mind being the Mature Face to show the efficacy of their wrinkle removing product. And when I told them no, because I definitely did not believe in chemical products, all over my face, and especially not theirs [this can show you that I am not very well known for my tact and diplomacy,] they were rather surprised. How could a supposedly cosmopolitan, supposedly well-educated and With It supposedly sophisticated human being leading an active social life, go out without using their world-famous global products as make-up?

When they sadly considered the alternative deciding that I was not working on all 24 cylinders, let me admit the reason why I have a wrinkle free complexion. That is because I definitely do not apply chemicals on my face. The only time I touch my face is when I am washing it with a natural oatmeal scrub – applied before a shower – and then moisturizing it with a mixture of honey and water.

If a wrinkle turns up eventually, as it is going to do as my skin loses its elasticity and collagen, I am not going to lose my head over it. Do you know that stress and tension is one of the main reasons why more and more people "feel" that they are growing old?

And one of the reasons why women are more conscious about the small wrinkle appearing here and there is because they are very particular about their looks. So, instead of growing old gracefully and accepting the fact that the skin is also going to grow old, and begin to show its age sometime or the other in their lives, they keep looking for chemical remedies which promise them everlasting youth.

These chemical remedies may make you look deceptively young, for a little while, but your skin is going to go back to its aged state, within a little while.

So I would suggest drinking plenty of fresh juice to keep your body well hydrated. A dehydrated body is going to show up more wrinkles. Also, do not go upon fussing with your face and body, with massages, lotions, potions and expensive makeovers. You may look good temporarily, but as the effect begins to wear off, you are going to look 50 again.

Tips for a Healthy, Youthful Skin

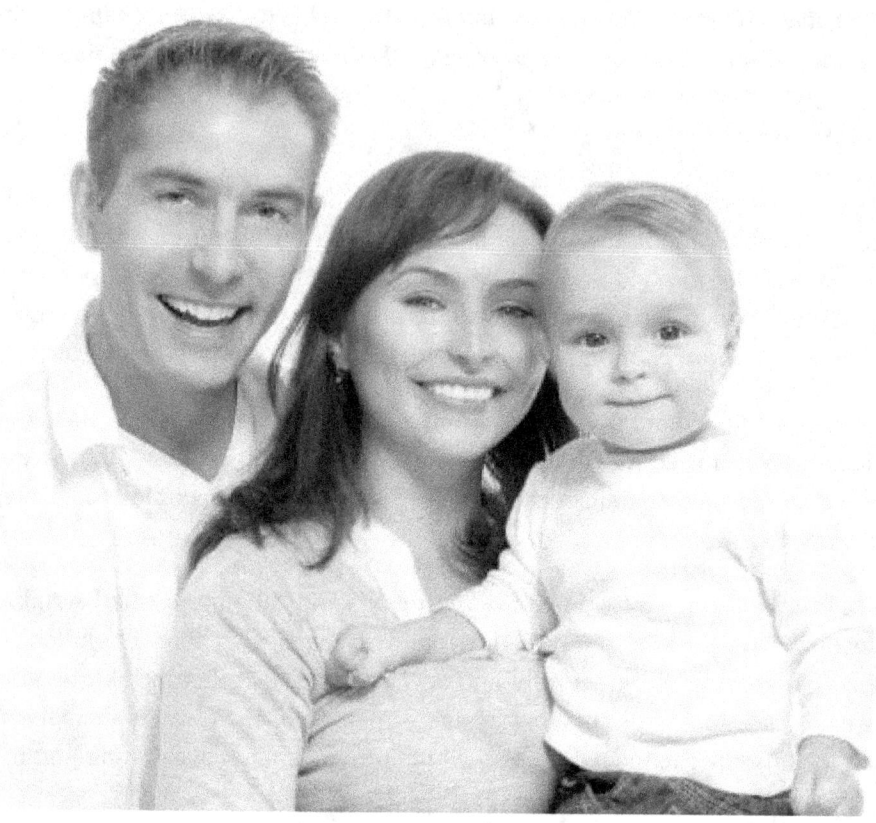

Keep out of the sun, as far as possible. Men may look handsome tanned, but the texture of their skin is different. Besides, they do not mind being sunburned. But if you are sunburned, remember that it is going to take anywhere between 6 to 12 months for your skin to get back to its original state of creaminess, unless of course it was a severe sunburn. And then you have had it.

If the skin has burnt so badly, down the superficial epidemic level to the endoderm is, it may probably never heal itself and you are going to have black sunburn patches all over your face and body.

Cabbage and Yeast

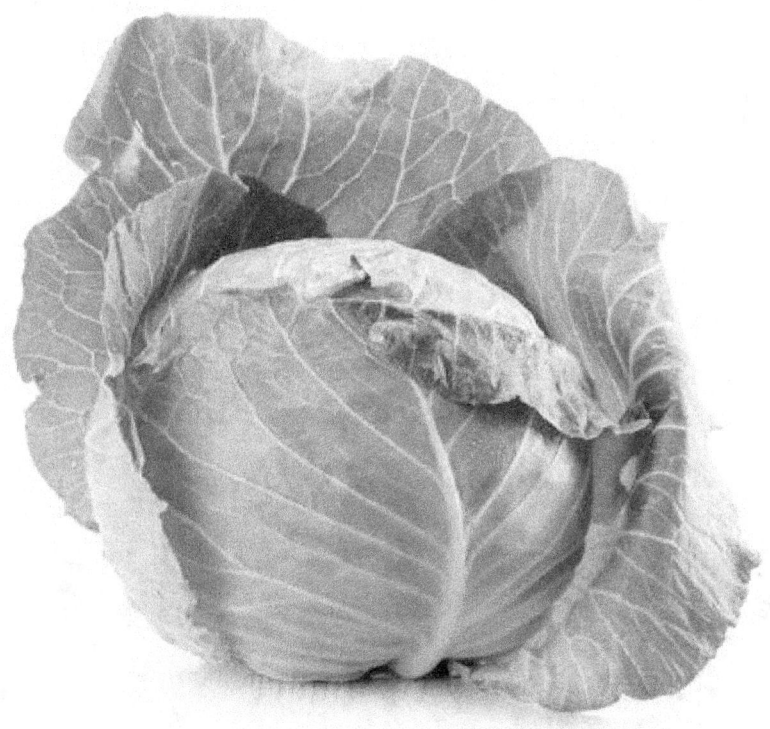

A wrinkle free skin can be obtained by dissolving one teaspoonful of yeast in one teaspoonful of cabbage juice and one tablespoonful of honey. Apply this paste all over your wrinkles, avoiding the eye region. Use this regularly to have a healthy wrinkle free skin.

Cabbage juice has been used down the ages to keep wrinkles at bay all over the world. Honey is of course a good moisturizer, as well as an antiseptic. Yeast can be considered to be a good rejuvenator, especially encouraging the cells of your skin to stay healthy and multiply in a proper glowing fashion.

Ice water Treatment

You can also oil your face with your favorite oil and then either move a cube of ice or wash your face with ice water. This is an excellent way to smoothen wrinkles.

Detoxification Diet

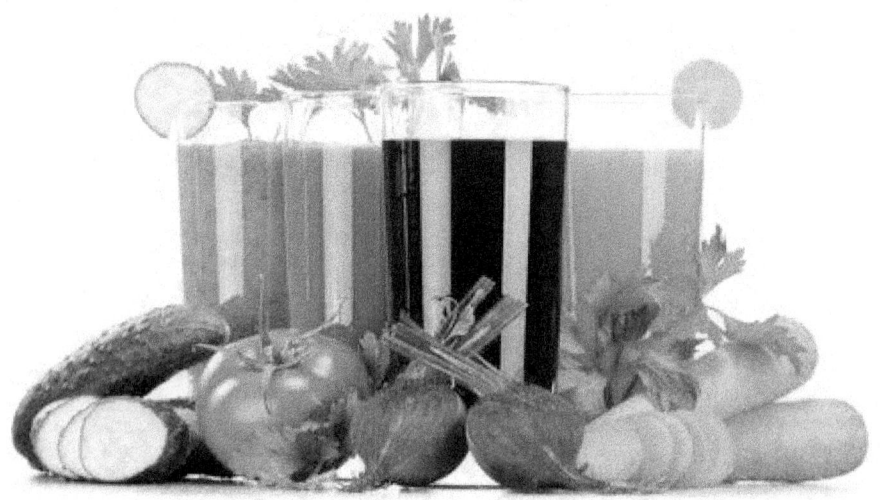

Try out a one-day diet where you are going to eat fruit, vegetables and water, and nothing else. Not only is this excellent to detoxify your body, but it is also going to have a good effect on your skin, especially if you decide to make it a 2 day diet.

Remember to take a cod liver pill daily. This is good for your immunity system. This is also good for general health.

I remember finding a bottle of old cod liver pills as a child. They looked so attractive, all golden in color. What I did not know that they were about 10 years old and the outer covering capsule had become all rubbery. And there I was, biting into one of those attractive pills, and getting a taste of very strong pepper.

For years afterwards, I associated that peppery taste with the original taste of or liver oil and would not touch it. Until somebody dared me to try one out and I found that The Seven Seas cod liver oil pills were rather good.

Well, this can be considered to be one of the good food items which I ate in abundance during childhood, and which gave me energy, as well as a good immunity system on a long-term basis.

Carrot Juice

Thanks to Walt Disney, all of us believe that carrot juice can improve our sight and make us see in the dark, because after all, Bugs Bunny has really sharp eyesight, especially when he is on his wascally wabbit antics.

There does not seem to be any real proof that carrot juice can improve eyesight, even though Beta carotene is extremely good for the body. So any juice which keeps your body healthy is good, do not you think.

Apart from drinking this carrot juice, you can apply the pulp of this carrot, along with carrot juice and honey to your face to smoothen out the wrinkles.

Rice Powder Treatment

This is the wrinkle smoothener recipe being used down the ages in areas of the east, where Rice is grown in abundance. So instead of oatmeal, or wheat bran, of course they use rice powder. Just apply a mixture of rice powder and honey on the wrinkles, and allow the mixture to dry. Then rub it off gently with warm water, in motions towards the heart.

Wash with warm water and apply a mixture of honey and water to help the skin regain its lost elasticity.

How to Use Honey and Water

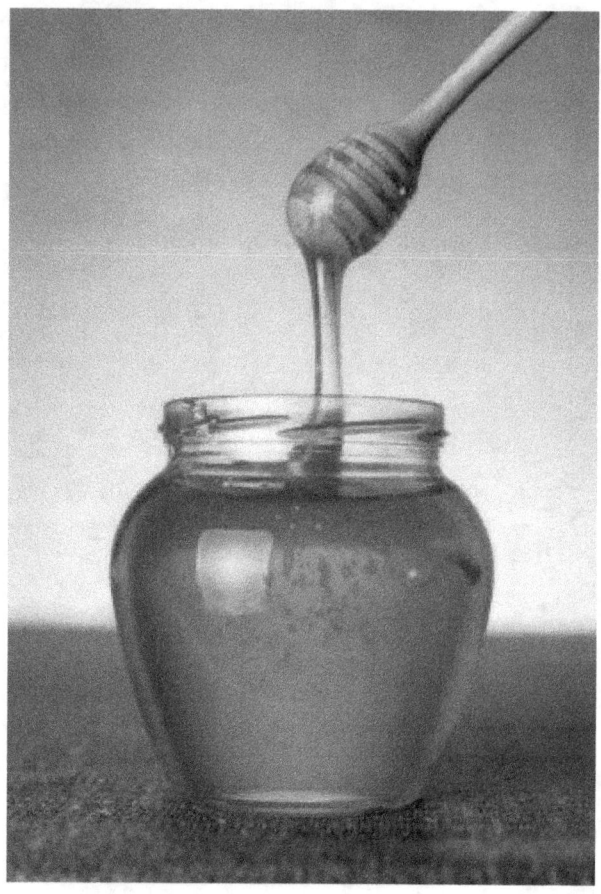

Many people do not apply honey to their face and body, because, well, honey is so sticky and icky. But here is a good way in which you are not going to feel the clammy stickiness of honey, especially during the summer.

Just pour some honey in a small bowl. Have another bowl full of ice water ready at hand. Dip a couple of fingers in the honey and then dip those fingers in the icewater. Apply it all over the skin in its diluted form.

One of Dame Barbara Cartland's well-known Toast of Society friends [Barbara herself was a very firm advocate and fan of pure honey for health and beauty] had this habit of going to sleep every afternoon with honey spread all over her face and neck. I am definitely not going to advocate it, because that means you are going to have sticky sheets and ants deciding that you are their best friends.

However, nobody stops you from applying pure honey – without any dilution – on the exposed parts of your body, especially those portions which are not going to come in contact with clothes, during the day. This honey is going to protect your skin as well as keep it healthy and moisturized.

Skin Snacks for Your Body

Believe it or not, your body would also like skin snacks. After all, it may be covered with dust and grime, and not get enough of water in order to keep it well hydrated. So give it, this nourishing the skin snack in order to moisturize, hydrate, as well as soften it.

One of my favorite skin snacks includes the white of an egg, along with my favorite oil, and one teaspoonful of apple cider vinegar. After that I put in one tablespoonful of yogurt and one tablespoonful of honey into this mixture and allow my skin to luxuriate in this nourishing snack.

This is going to wash off in the shower, so I normally apply it about an hour before showering. The vinegar and the honey and the oil is going to soak in, while the yogurt and the dried white is going to be rubbed off, leaving my skin silky smooth and healthy.

Best Night Time Skin Lotion/Moisturizer/Cleanser

This is the only time when I am asking you to use a product which is not hundred percent natural – glycerin. But then I found this glycerin as an excellent skin tonic base.

Take equal parts of glycerin, Rosewater, almond oil, (you can also use wheat germ oil), and honey. Add the juice of one lemon to this rich, exotic and possibly expensive mixture. Wash your face with warm water, and then apply this lotion with a cotton bud all over your face.

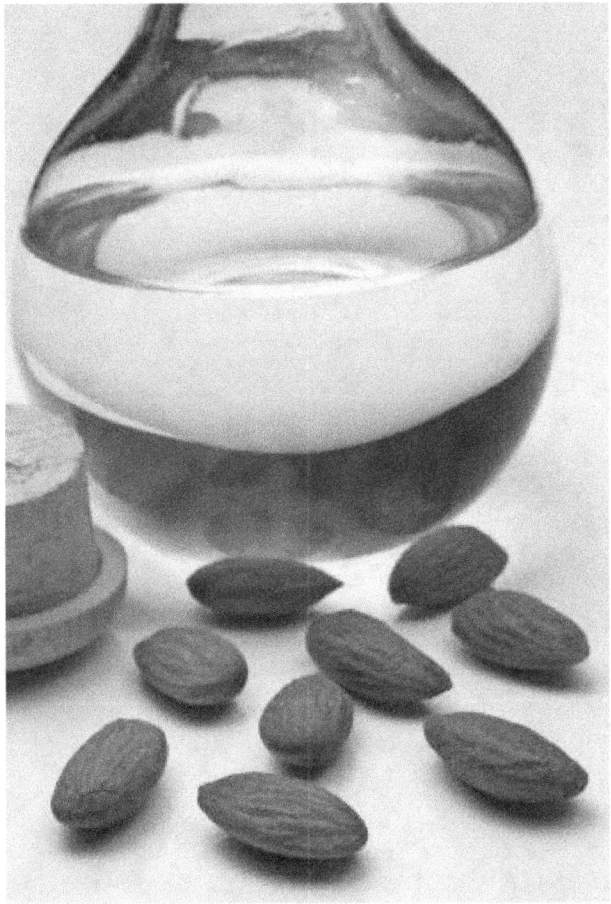

Marilyn Monroe went to bed wearing Chanel No 5. Well, that was her prerogative, because it was only once in my life that I made the mistake of putting a few drops of my mother's treasured *Magie Noir* into this lotion. I thought that it would impart a sweet smelling scent to my skin All Night Long.

Never again! The chemicals in the powerful perfume spoiled the whole natural balance of this lotion. Heavy and chemical perfumes do not have the seductive power of natural perfumes. If you really have to bring on the artillery, let it have the power of nature! If you want to add some natural perfume, try adding essential oils.

Patchy and Rough Skin

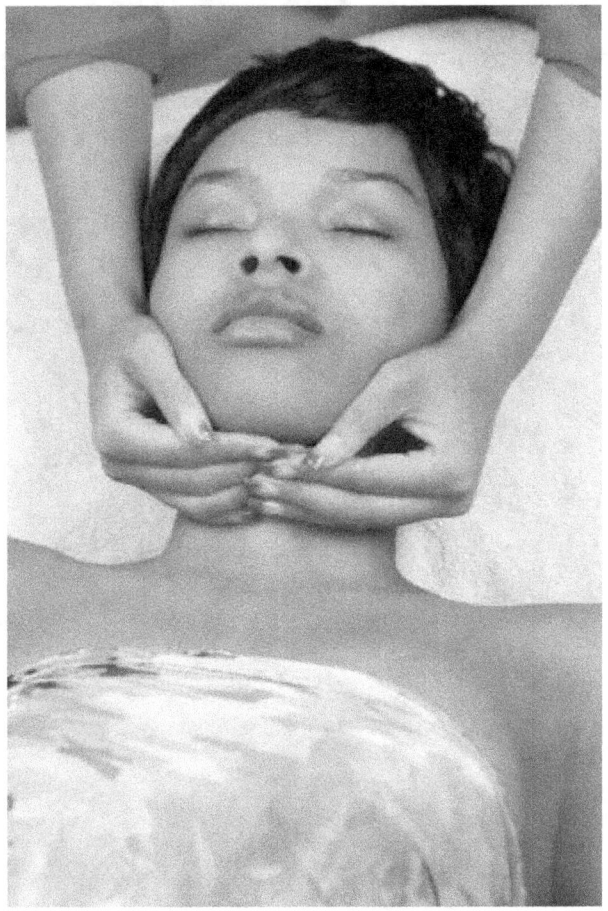

Good skin care means no rough skin…

Well, we have a tendency of neglecting the skin of our elbows and ankles can also be smoothened out, softened and whitened.

Make a paste of five tablespoons rice flour, five tablespoons sour yogurt and half a teaspoon of turmeric. Add a thick layer on the areas you want to treat and leave it for 10 minutes till the paste is dry. Rub off the paste with warm water. A regular application soon smoothens out the rough patches.

The glycerin and lemon juice lotion is best for bringing your skin to its normal and natural color.

Now there are two types of making infused oils, the sun method or the working lady method! The slow sun method is for that lady, who has a beautiful garden with lots of sunlight streaming in. The working lady method is, of course, for the lady who does not have time to breathe and as she is working on a tight time schedule, wants everything done yesterday! (You know, my sort, always looking for shortcuts done everywhere, so this can be done best on a Sunday!)

Rosewater

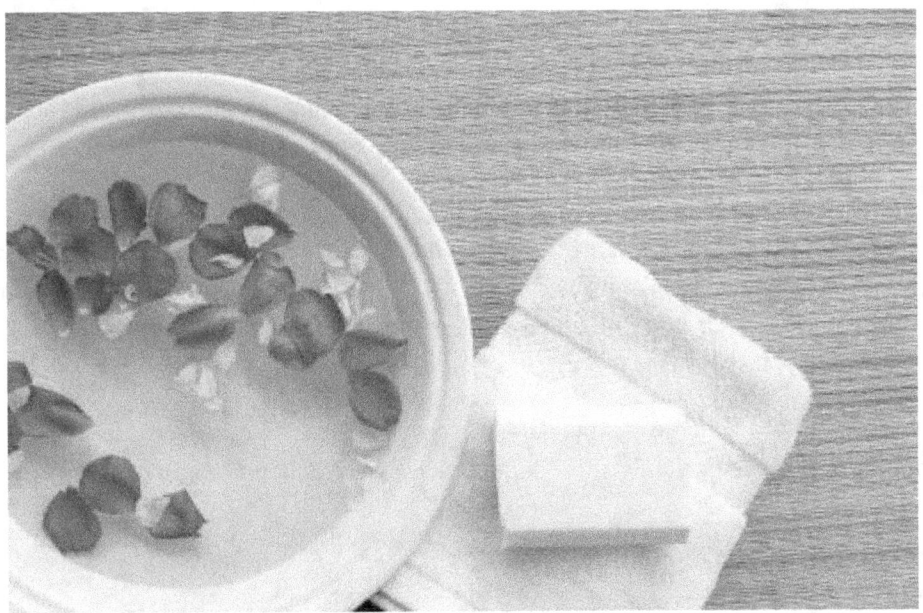

Rosewater is an essential beauty ingredient, which is made from red roses. Four millenniums, beauties in the East have been using this ingredient as one way in which to keep their skins healthy, nourished and well bleached. This is also a nice perfume, which gives a rose fragrance to your skin.

If you have plenty of time and energy, and you happen to live in an area which is very sunny you can make Rosewater through the –

Slow Sun Method

I normally choose a light vegetable oil like sunflower oil, but my grandmother used to infuse herbs in ghee (Clarified butter – also known as desi ghee or native butter] or freshly homemade butter. I have noticed that the ghee infusions are more powerful, because of their concentrated power to heal.

 But then everybody knows my always To Let pockets would screech blue murder if I spent lots of money on pure and expensive desi ghee, just for the sole purpose of using it in infusions instead of eating it and so gaining full value for my money , so if you do have a good supply of homemade desi ghee , be my guest and use it !

Anyway, collect your flower petals -- red roses please , the ones which are so popular in making garlands and bouquets – they are called Damascus Rose.

Then, fill a large glass jar   with a good vegetable oil, or homemade butter or ghee.

Add the rose petals until they are covered with the oil but are not tightly packed, (I found out that three -- 4 handfuls of the petals did me just fine, there was enough of space for all of them to breathe.)

Cover with an air tight lid and leave in direct sunshine. The rose petals will turn brown after a couple of days. Remove them and add fresh blooms. Repeat this procedure until the oil is tinged pink. (The more changes you do, the more you have rose extract in the oil in your precious bottle.)

People in the East are very lucky because they have a good supply of rose flowers as well as direct sunlight, but in many the Western countries tough luck when all ye sun deprived people have to go up to 20 or more changes because of the uncertain summer season and rainy weather.

The more you persevere, and the more patient you are, the more this rather long method captures the fragrance of the delicate flower.

The second method is the-

Quick Kitchen Method:

To make *gulabjal* (rose water) and extract essential oils from herbs . Buying it in the market, especially when it is marketed as a very exotic beauty ingredient from the East may turn out to be expensive. So make it yourself.

For this method, you need to have a large supply of petals , and lots of ice handy!

Take a large cooking pot, insert a clean brick or rock in its bottom , fill the pot with rose petals , the more the merrier, or herbs around the brick. Cover with water and place a small glass dish on top of the brick.

On top of the pot put a stainless steel bowl and fill with ice. Simmer about three hours depending how many petals or herbs you have, replacing the ice as needed. The bowl with the ice will condense the steam which will then drip down into the glass bowl. The water in the glass bowl is your rose water or whatever herb, on top will be a layer of oil. This is the essential oil.

You can separate these and use the water in cooking, or as *Gulab jal* and the essential oil in lotions, soaps or whatever.

And this is the precious extract, which is sold in the market for 80 $ every 10 g! And even then, it is not the real thing, because it has been adulterated with geranium oil. It takes up to 60,000 roses to extract 1 ounce of oil so could you wonder why it comes under the most rare and expensive of oils.

This rosewater is one of the most essential commodities of every self-respecting and enterprising beauty conscious lady's beauty arsenal. Not only does this moisturize the skin and keep it silky and soft, but it also imparts a soft scented fragrance, which is more appealing than the heavy musky and expensive parfums, which are alas, so often a regular and cloying substitute for neglected ablutions.

Method Two

For this, you will have to have all the petals as well as a vegetable oil ready. 1 1/2 cups of vegetable oil and 250 grams of petals gave me 1 1/2 cups of infused oil.

Place half of the rose petals and all the oil in a container with a tight lid.

Put a container in a pan, fill the pan up with water to within 1 inch of the top of the container and simmer this slowly for 2 hours. This water bath makes sure that your precious oil is exposed to prolonged heating without spoiling the oil by burning or boiling. To save time and energy costs, I normally boil 2-3 airtight containers together.

After two hours, allow the mixture to cool slightly and then strain it well. Now, we are just halfway through the process and the infusion has changed color. At this strength, this infusion is mild enough to use as baby oil or bath oil. Refill the canister with the remaining rose petals , cover with the strained oil and return to the water bath.

Simmer gently for another two hours. Don't forget to replace the lid! Also make sure to check the water level to make sure that the water has not boiled away completely. Nobody has any use for burnt oil.

When the oil has cooked enough, pour it through a muslin cloth or very fine strainer. If you are using fresh petals, there might be some watery liquid at the bottom of the oil. Remember to separate out this liquid and throw it away, because it is quite certain to spoil the oil if it is left unattended to.

Once the oil has been strained , gather all the petals in the cloth and wring them out to extract every drop of oil . This oil will keep fresh for a year but it will eventually become rancid. Many cosmetologists thus add some wheat germ oil to delay the spoiling process -- (about 25 g.)

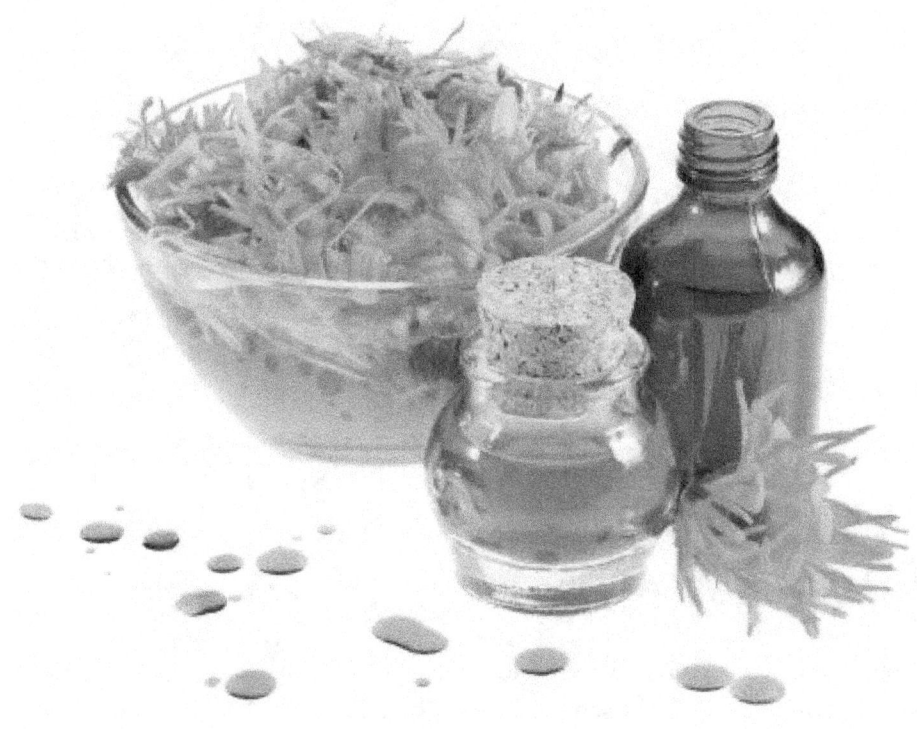

Marigold essential oil and marigold water is also made the same way as Rose water.

As for the spent petals, I do not throw them away, but I put them into my bathwater so as not to waste them! These oils have to be poured into clean bottles. Remember to store them away in dark and not transparent bottles in a cool and dark place away from the sunlight.

Sprinkle your skin with Rosewater lavishly, whenever you think your skin feels dry. This is the best cooling natural liquid ever known to man.

Giving Luster to Your Skin

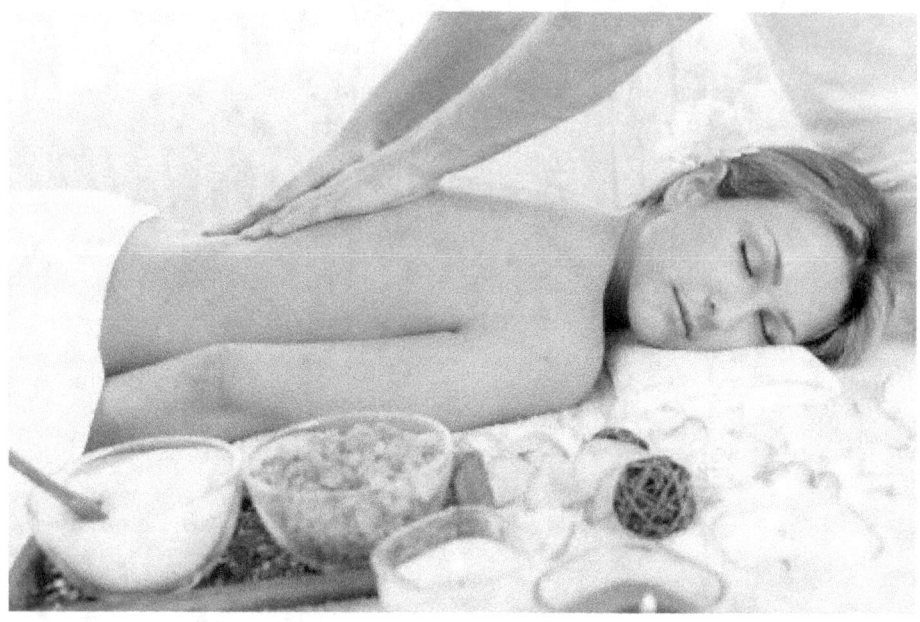

A massage is an excellent way which you can tone up your skin. Make sure that only natural oils are used for massaging

Coconut oil and almond oil are excellent for massaging purposes. Bob Hope once wrote about traveling with a famous Italian superstar, who settled herself in the plane and took out a bottle of olive oil. And then, she slowly and steadily began to massage the oil into her body, during the flight.

According to Mr. Hope, and which I think an exaggeration, by the time the flight was done, the bottle was also done. But again, there are people who could think of massaging a whole bottle of olive oil into their skin, during a forty-five minute flight. But then Ms. Lolobrigida - a runner up in a Miss Italia contest – was known for her exquisite skin. She worked on keeping it so.

If you are massaging the oil, in your body, make sure that you are doing so with the tips of your fingers in light circular motions, towards your heart. Massaging with your hand does not have that light touch, except if the skin is being pummeled and punched.

Skin Bleachers

Believe it or not, one of the most popular items in the billion-dollar beauty industry is skin bleachers of every kind. These bleaching creams are very much in demand, because marketing strategies throughout the years have instilled it in the minds of many people that a bleached and fair skin automatically makes one more attractive and lovely.

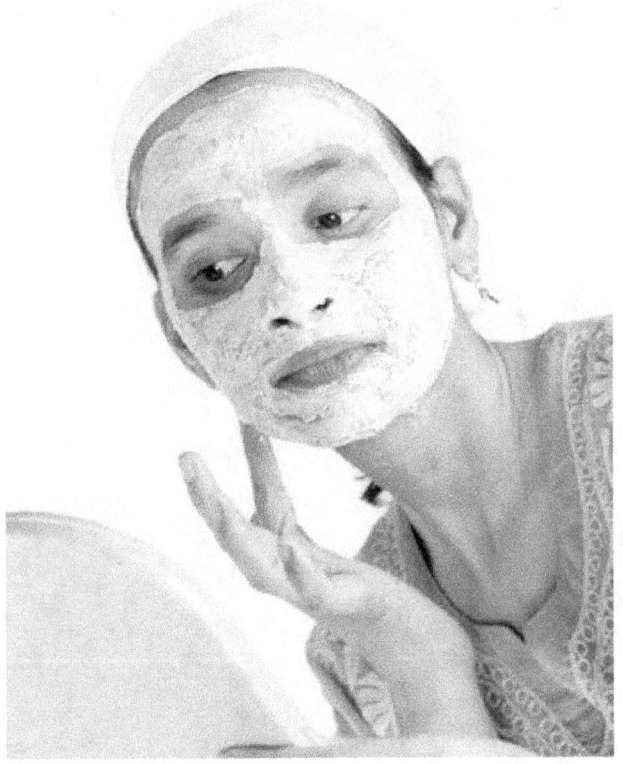

Basically, I would not mind a bit of suntan, but since childhood, it was drilled into our collective psyches, that as we were born with comparatively fair skins, it was our bound duty to preserve and protect them.[1] So is it surprising that when a person grows into an adult, he automatically reaches for the nearest bleaching cream, the moment he finds himself just this little bit dusky brown.

So, naturally, here are some bleaching recipes which you may want to try out. Incidentally, this recipe was given to me by a Scandinavian friend, who is, of course, as peaches and cream as the driven snow, being a blonde beauty. Nevertheless, she wants to bleach her skin even more. Go figure. For this, she used a nightly mixture of salt and fresh milk on her skin to rub off the dust and grime, as well as bleach out the skin.

But well, so did her grandmother and her grandmother before her, and possibly that is why Nordic beauties have been known for their good looks down the ages.

---

[11] - That meant that the girl would grow up to be "Fair and Lovely" – this term spoken in a rush like ham and eggs, Laurel and Hardy and so on. Fairness is still equated with attractiveness in many parts of the East, especially in girls.

Orange Peel

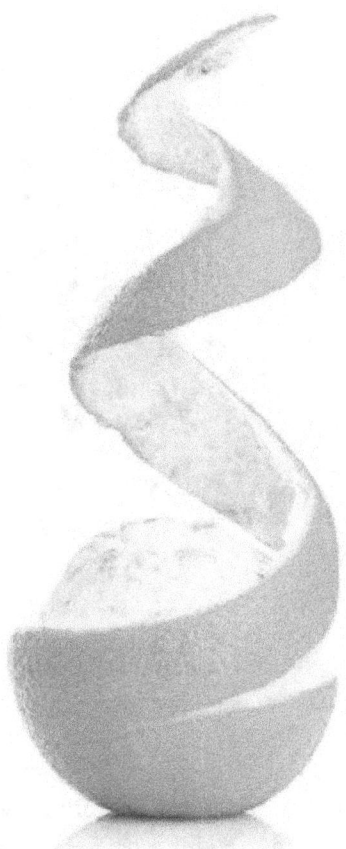

Orange peel has been well-known as an excellent skin bleacher for centuries. Just take some dried orange peels, and make them into a powder. Put it in an airtight jar for future use. Take one tablespoonful of this peel, and make a mixture with milk.

Use this as a face scrub, by applying it on your face, and leaving on for twenty-five minutes. That is the amount of time it takes for the orange peel to dry, before you can rub it off with warm water. Use this daily. Believe it or not, your skin will start bleaching out within fifteen days. That is unless the melanin content is genetically very high, and you come by your dark skin naturally.

Almond Bleacher

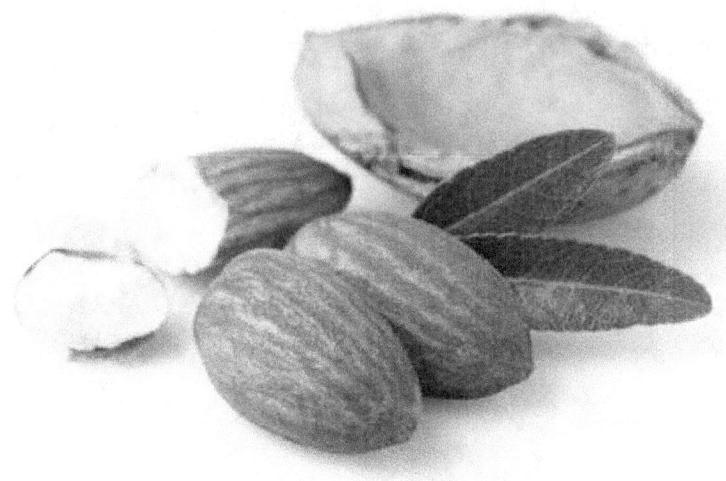

Almonds have been used for centuries as a natural bleacher, especially in the Middle East where beauties knew everything about natural beauty products down the ages.

For this, you need one teaspoonful of yogurt, +1 tablespoon full of oats and one tablespoonful of powdered almonds. Make a paste and apply it on your suntanned skin. Apply regularly and see the change in your skin texture as well as your skin bleaching out.

To tell you very frankly, I was analyzing this particular bleaching out recipe, and I decided that it was not the almonds so much as the yogurt which was the culprit.

Any milk product like cream and yogurt, and raw milk has been known down the centuries to be extremely powerful and amazing bleaching products.

Natural Bleaching Cream

This is a traditional natural bleaching cream, which was told to me by one of my beautician friends. Believe it or not, she does not use any of the beauty products marketed in the market, even though she uses them with great success on her clients. Rather, she would prefer natural products to be applied on her skin. Talk about double standards!

So if you want to get rid of blemishes on your skin, or bleach it, add a little bit of powdered oatmeal/wheat bran/chickpea flour – also known as *besan-*, three pinches of salt and a little bit of turmeric to 3 g lemon peel powder. Mix it in pure milk cream, put in a porcelain container and preserve it in your fridge.

Now before you go to sleep at night, you are going to rub your face, hands, arms and neck with this cleansing and bleaching mixture. Wash this off with warm water after 10 minutes.

This is an amazing skin toner, cleanser and natural bleacher. You may also find the blemishes on your skin disappearing. So if you want to appear really fair, try this bleaching and moisturizing cleanser.

Natural Hand Lotion

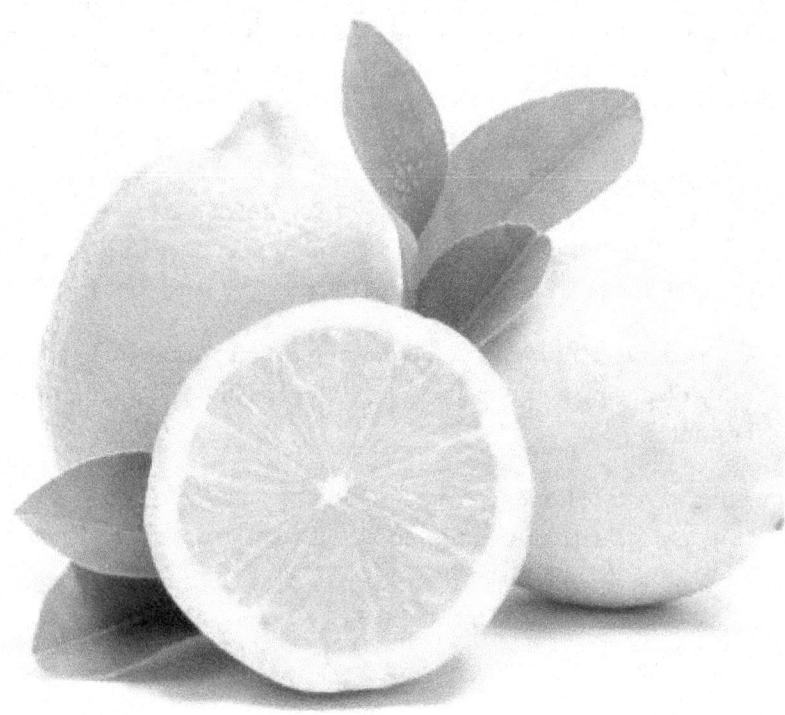

This is an excellent way to keep your hands soft and moisturized, especially when you feel that they are getting to be dishpan hands. This is the nursing and moisturizing skin lotion and that is why I normally use wheat germ or almond oil as moisturizers. This lotion is slightly sticky, so if you are applying it at bedtime, you might want to wash your hands before you drop off to sleep.

You may want to use it as a protective base under powder or makeup, if you pancake your face with chemicals throughout the day.

For this, you need two teaspoonful of lemon juice, and 2 teaspoons full of your favorite moisturizing oil. Mix the oil and the lemon juice very well until it is creamy. Apply immediately, rubbing in your hands to keep the skin moist, healthy and supple.

Protective Foot Powder

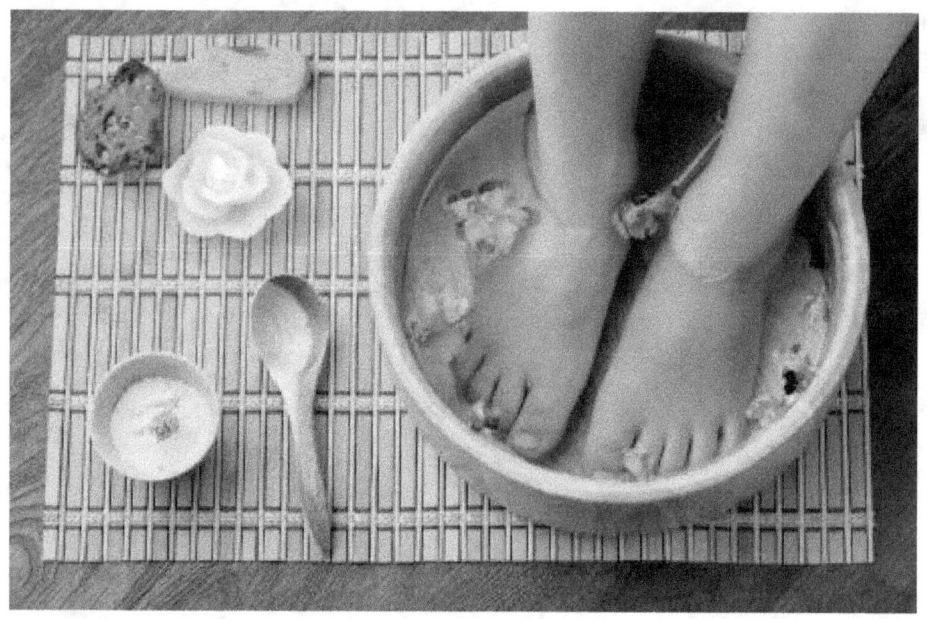

Soaking your feet in warm water with essential oils added is very refreshing.

 This powder can be made easily by taking one tablespoonful of cornstarch, one teaspoonful of bicarbonate of soda and one teaspoonful of herbs like parsley or thyme.

Mix all the ingredients together, and then sprinkle all over your well dried feet after a bath.

If you are suffering from athletes' foot, rub your feet to beforehand, with lemon peel. That is going to heal the fungal infection, thanks to the lemon's essential oil. Then sprinkle this foot powder all over your feet. These herbs are excellent in preventing skin infections, especially during the rainy season or when the atmosphere is moist and muggy.

Natural Deodorant

Thanks to our habit of sprinkling deodorants on, under clothes , made up of synthetic fibers, is it a wonder why so many of us fall prey to skin infections, especially in a humid atmosphere?

Here is a good natural deodorant which you can make by taking the rind of one lemon, a handful of rose petals, and a handful of mint leaves. Boil these three items together and leave overnight.

The next morning, filter it and bottle it. Use this natural deodorant instead of your expensive chemical-based deodorant from now on.

Conclusion

This book gives you plenty of information on skin and body care, especially with easily available ingredients. These recipes have been in use down the centuries, and are time-tested and time-honored. So take full advantage of this knowledge imparted down the ages and stay beautiful and youthful!

Live Long and Prosper!

Authors Bio

Dueep Jyot Singh is a Management and IT Professional who managed to gather Postgraduate qualifications in Management and English and Degrees in Science, French and Education while pursuing different enjoyable career options like being an hospital administrator, IT,SEO and HRD Database Manager/ trainer, movie , radio and TV scriptwriter, theatre artiste and public speaker, lecturer in French, Marketing and Advertising, ex-Editor of Hearts On Fire (now known as Solstice) Books Missouri USA, advice columnist and cartoonist, publisher and Aviation School trainer, ex- moderator on Medico.in, banker, student councilor ,travelogue writer, … among other things!

One fine morning, she decided that she had enough of killing herself by Degrees and went back to her first love -- writing. It's more enjoyable! She already has 48 published academic and 14 fiction- in- different- genre books under her belt.

When she is not designing websites or making Graphic design illustrations for clients , she is browsing through old bookshops hunting for treasures, of which she has an enviable collection – including R.L. Stevenson, O.Henry, Dornford Yates, Maurice Walsh, De Maupassant, Victor Hugo, Sapper, C.N. Williamson, "Bartimeus" and the crown of her collection- Dickens "The Old Curiosity Shop," and so on… Just call her "Renaissance Woman") - collecting herbal remedies, acting like Universal Helping Hand/Agony Aunt, or escaping to her dear mountains for a bit of exploring, collecting herbs and plants and trekking.

Our books are available at
1. Amazon.com
2. Barnes and Noble
3. Itunes
4. Kobo
5. Smashwords
6. Google Play Books

Check out some of the other JD-Biz Publishing books
Gardening Series on Amazon

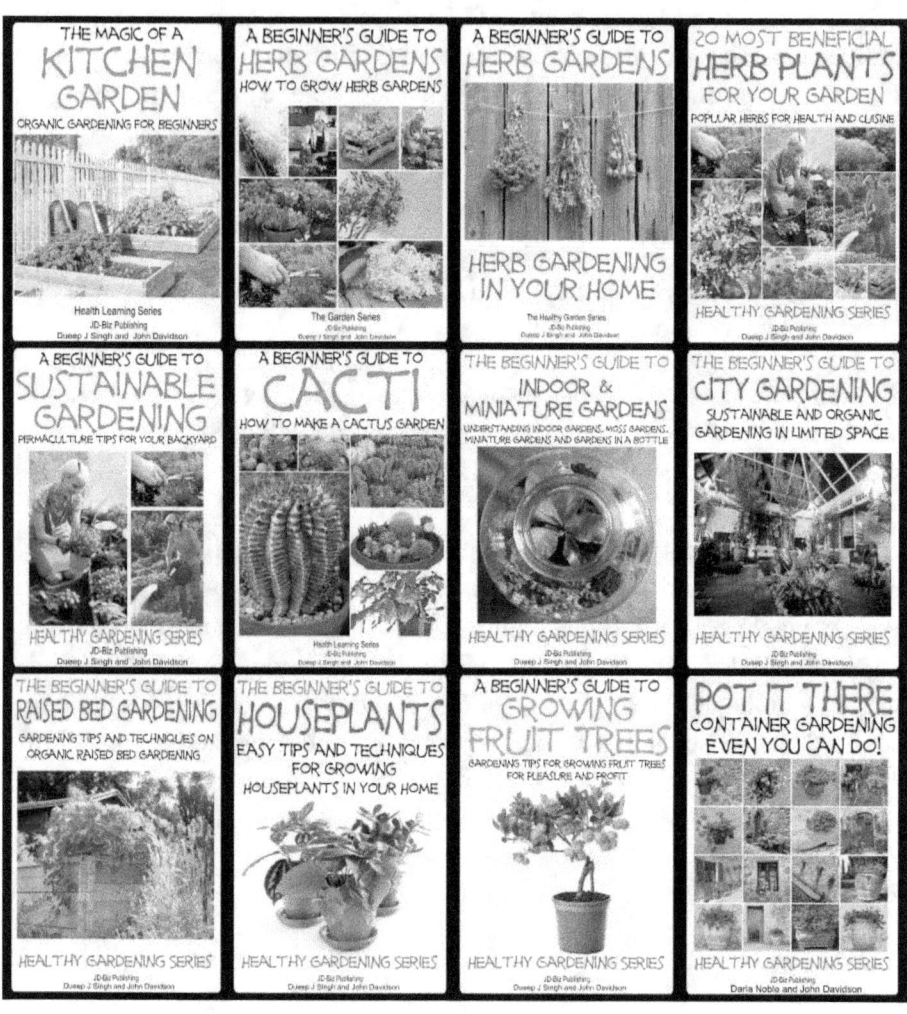

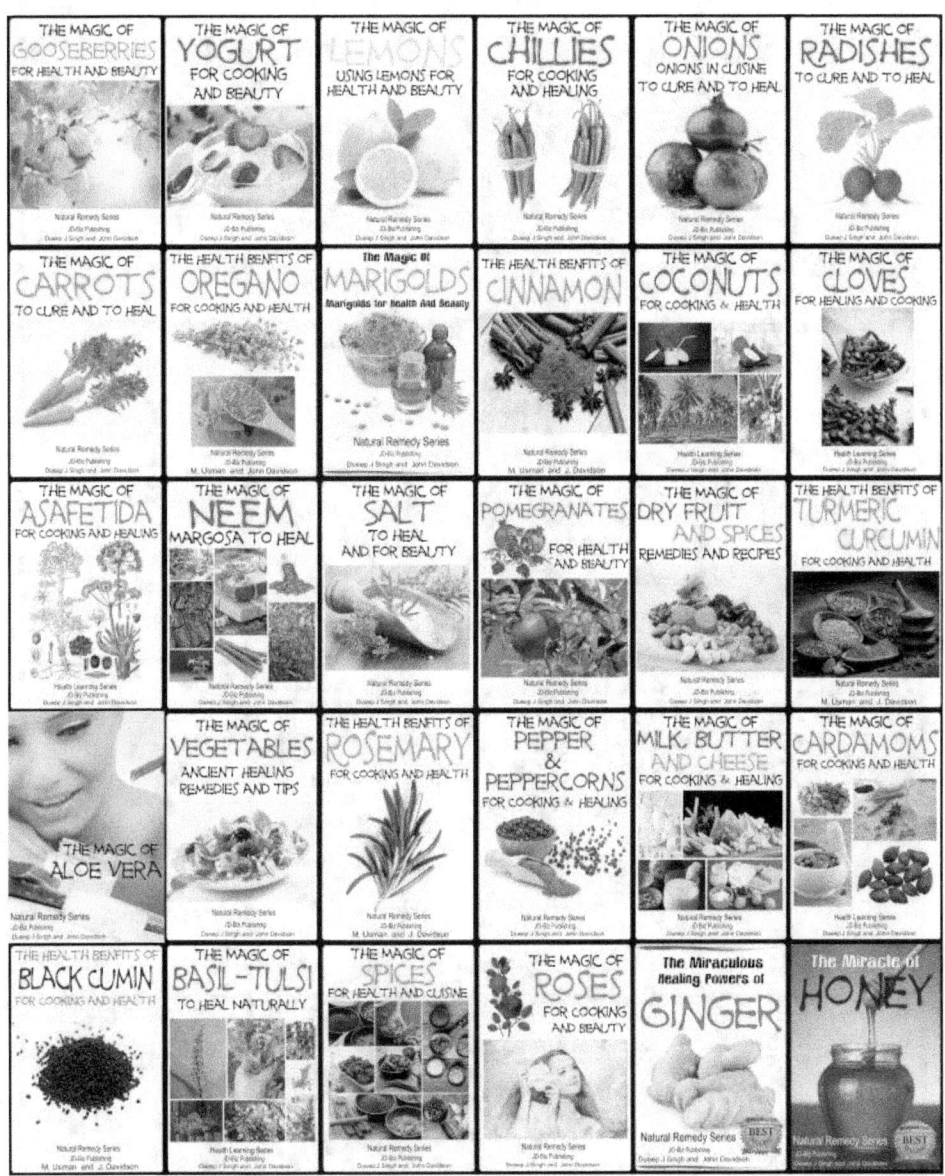

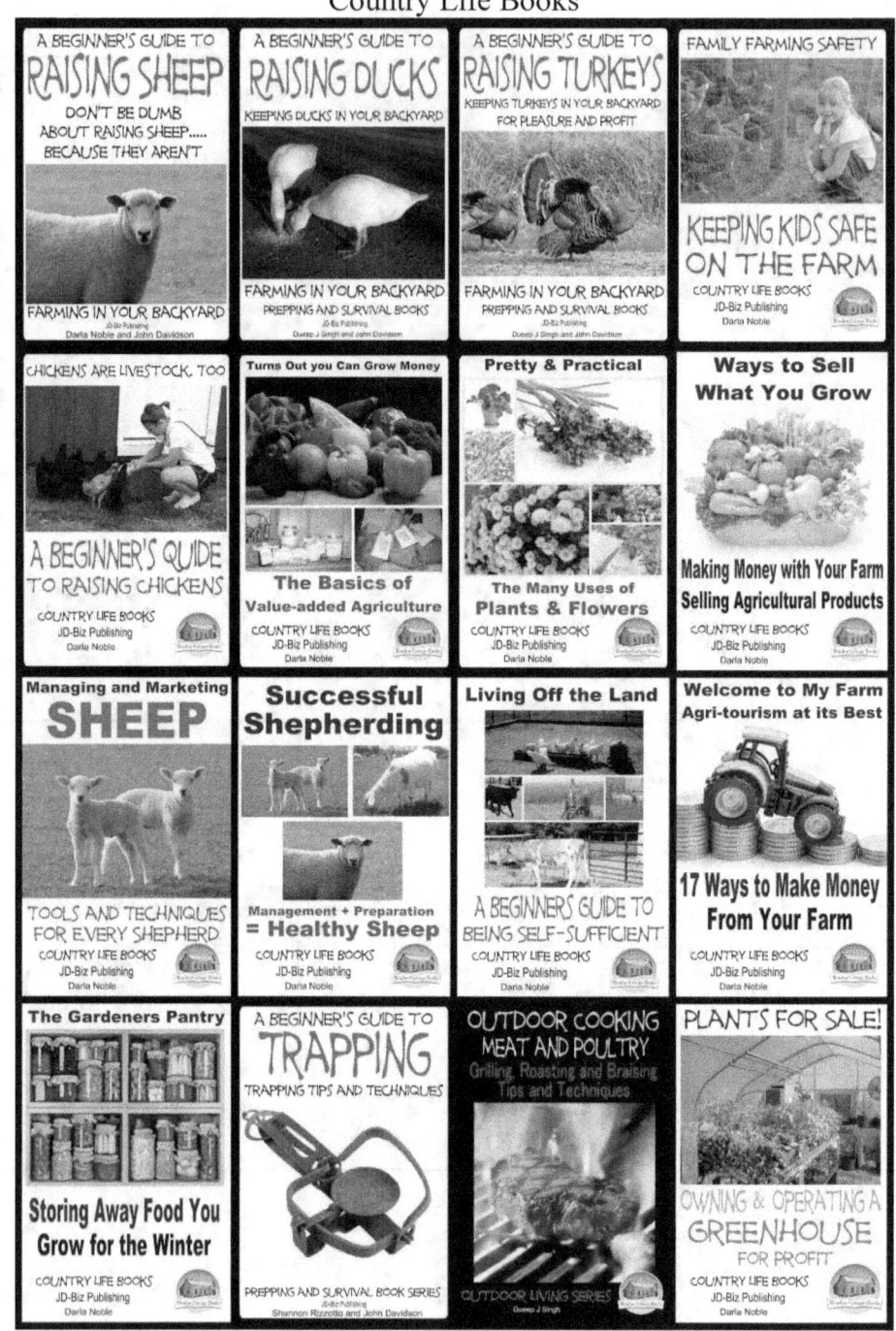

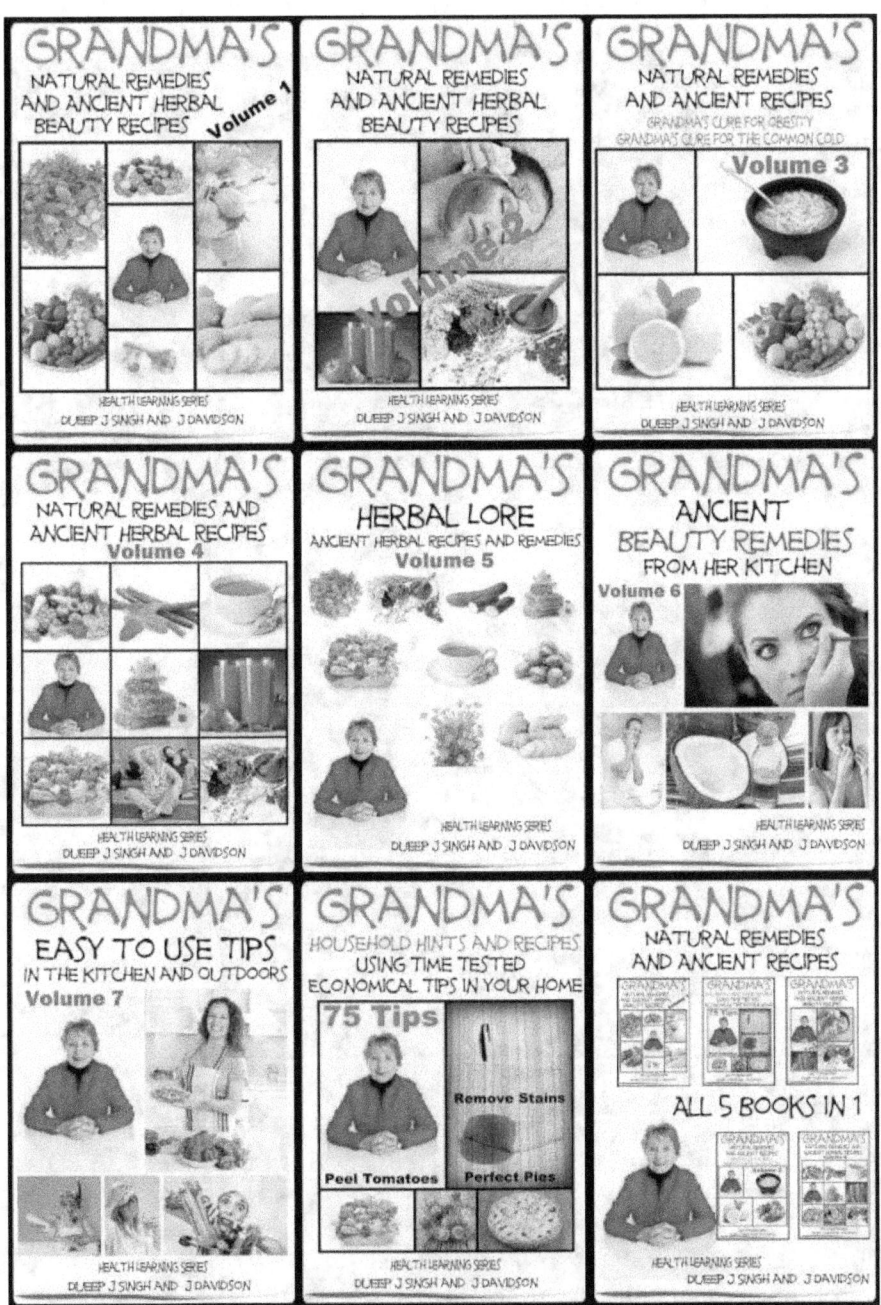

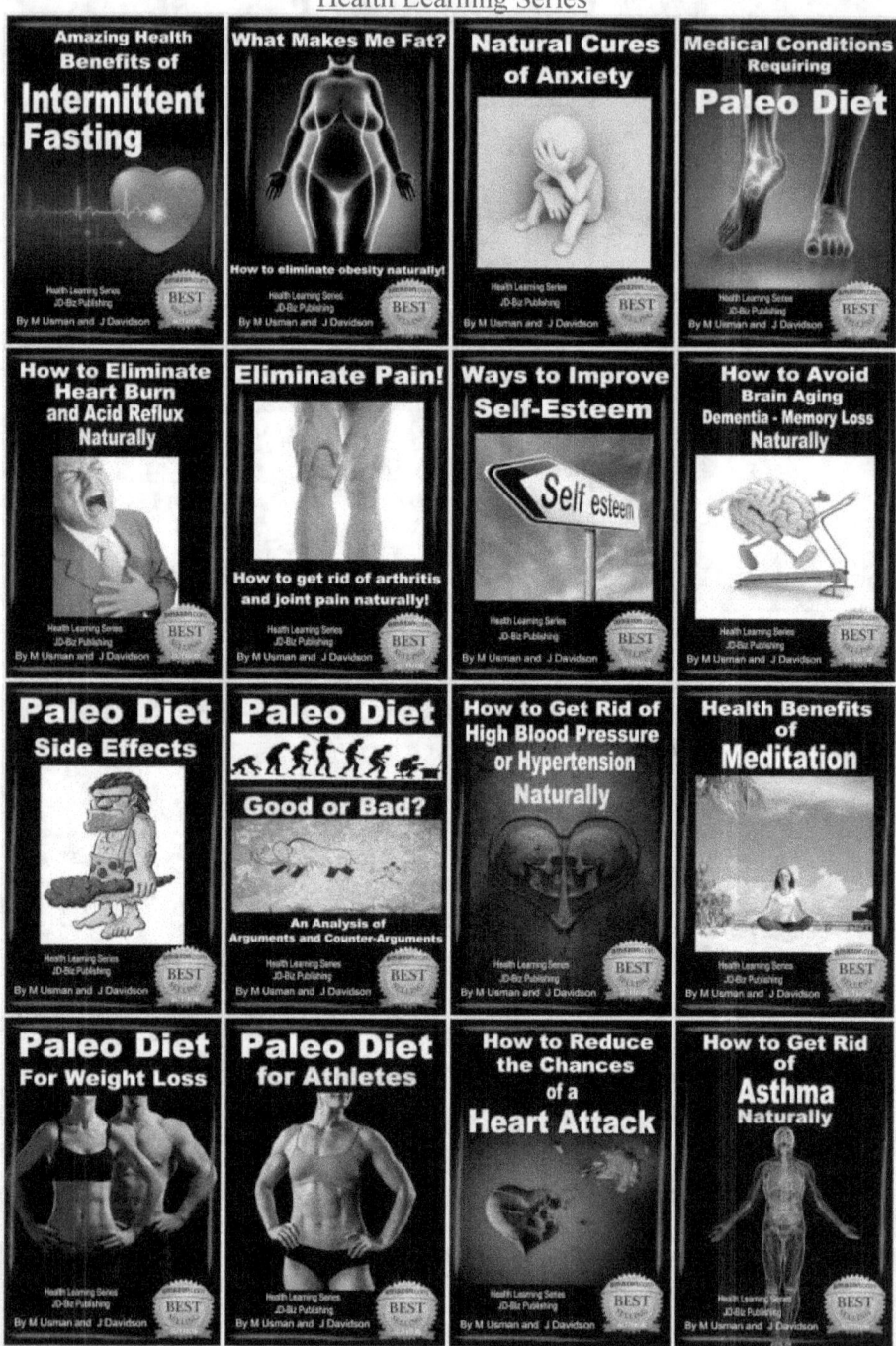

Amazing Animal Book Series

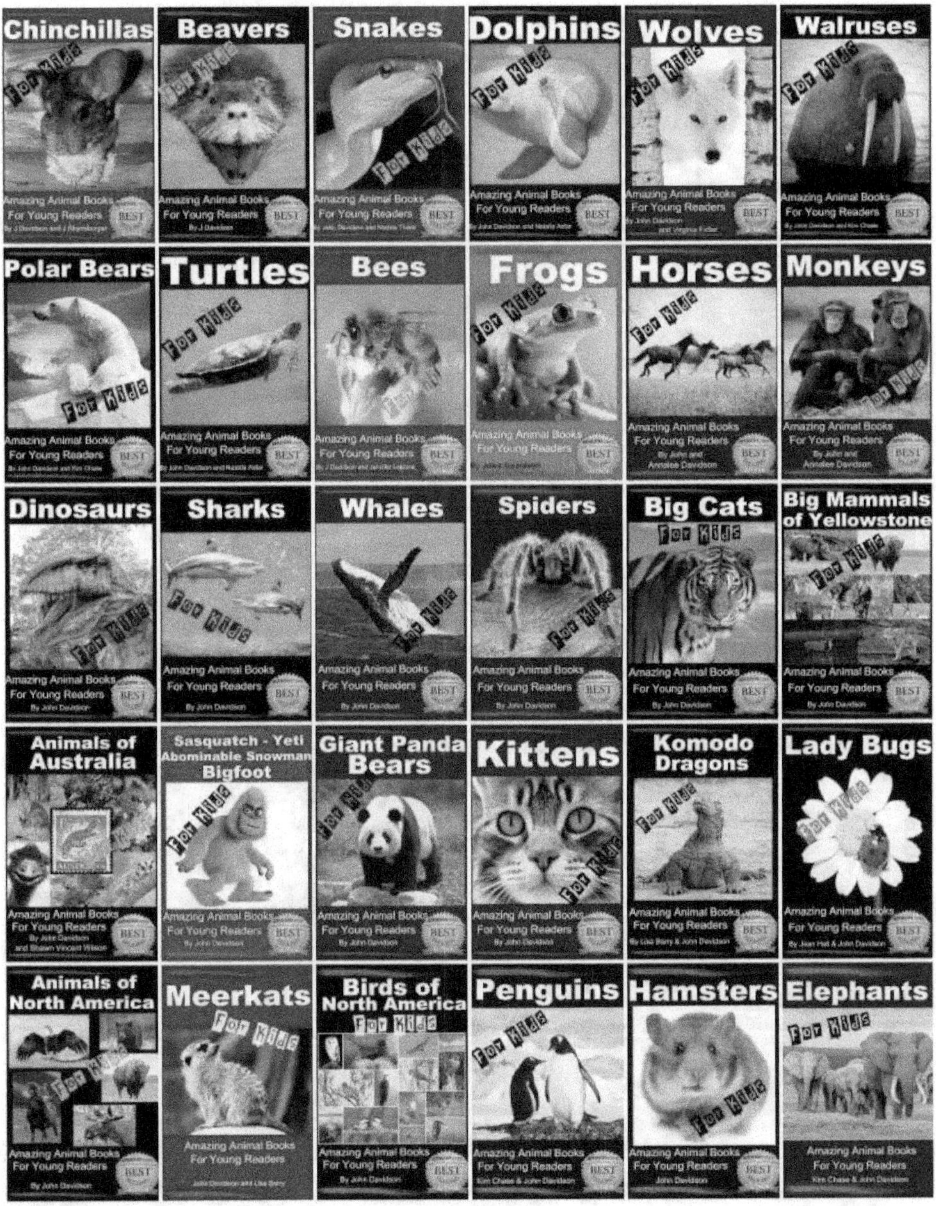

Learn To Draw Series

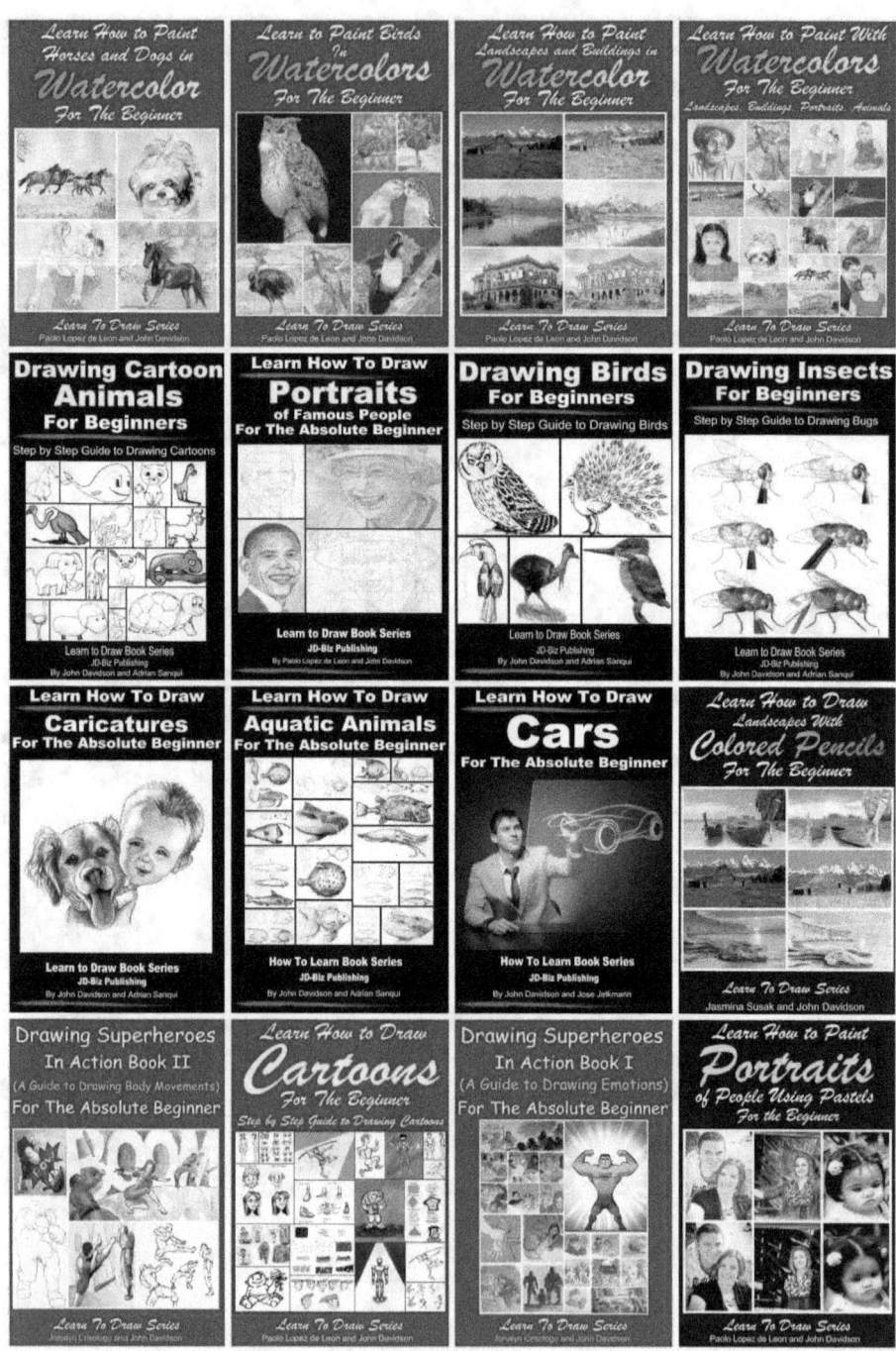

How to Build and Plan Books

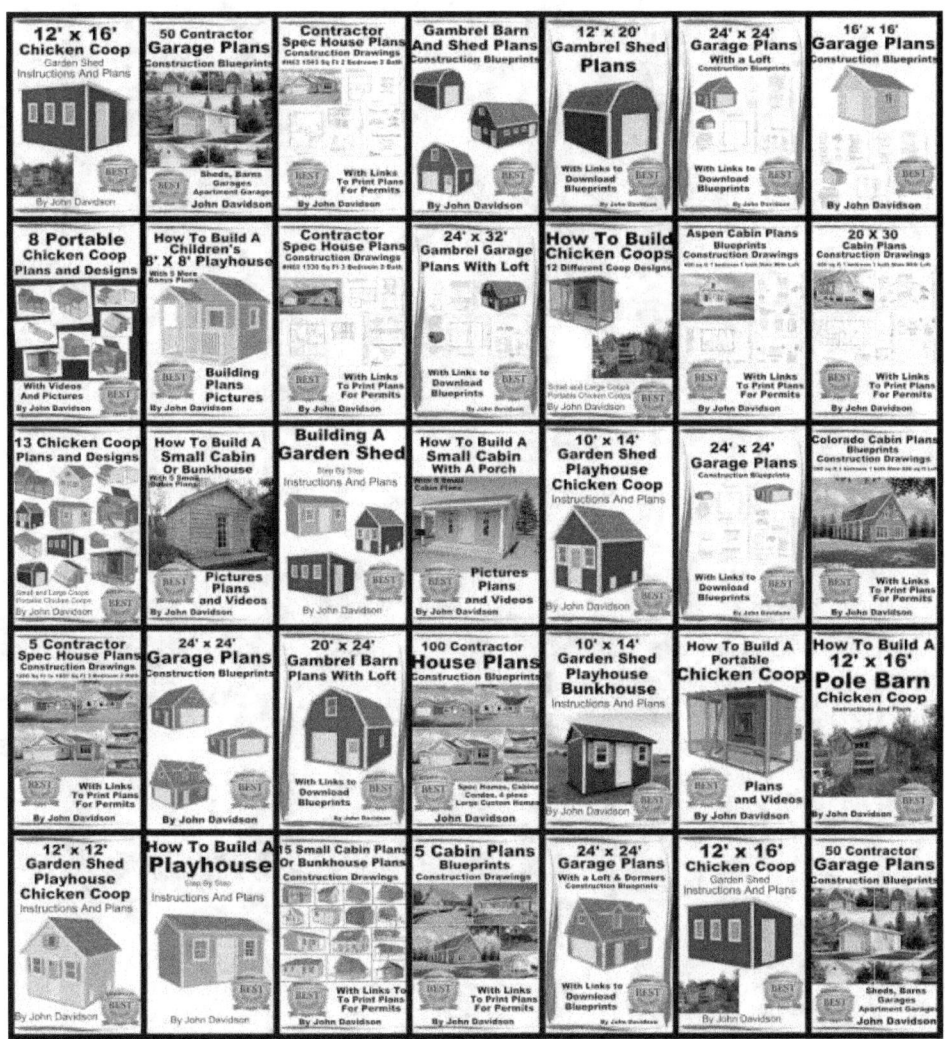

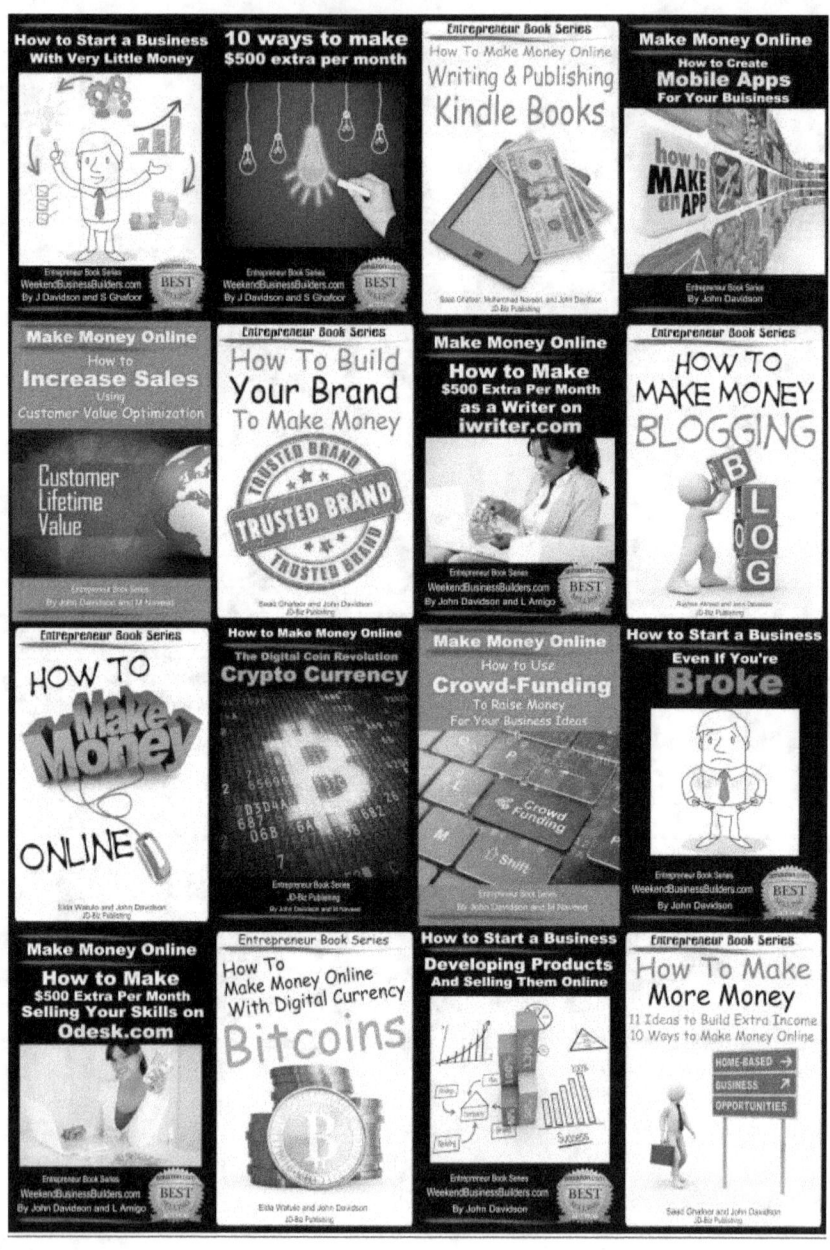

Publisher

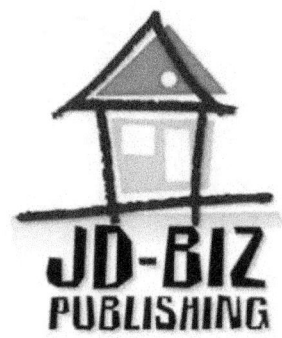

JD-Biz Corp

P O Box 374

Mendon, Utah 84325

http://www.jd-biz.com/

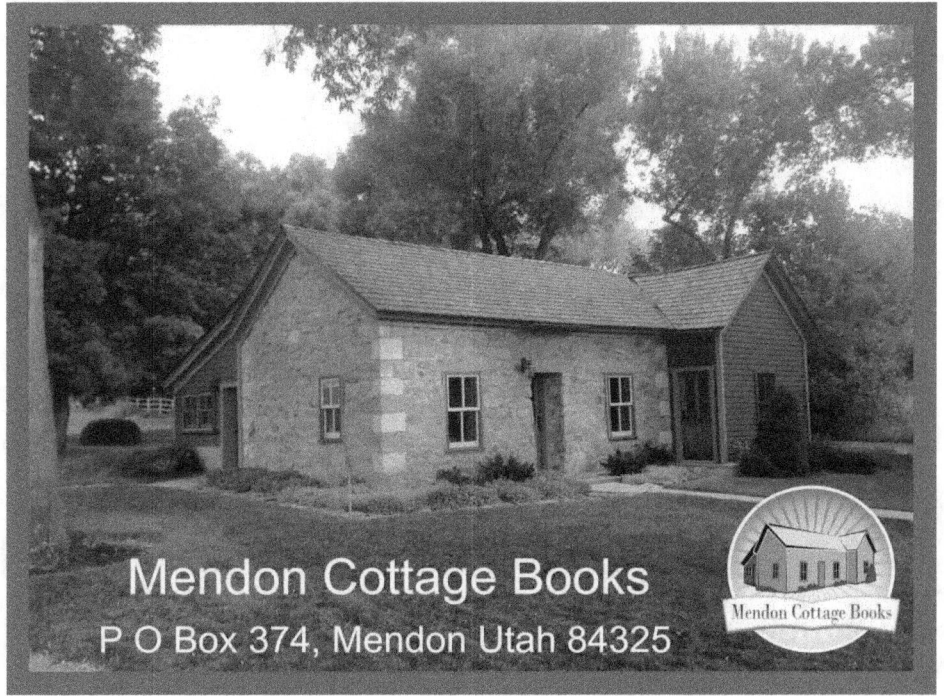